ISBN: 9798827634324

I0758130

Menopause Weight Loss Guide

How to Lose Weight Safely
and Effectively after 50

INTRODUCTION

Many women ask themselves "How to lose weight after 50?". If you are among them, you're not alone. With age, it becomes more challenging to lose weight. However, it is possible to achieve your weight loss goals and live a healthier, more fulfilling life when you take the right approach. The first thing you need to understand is that your body changes as you age and your metabolism slows down. In other words, you cannot eat like you did when you were young, and expect to lose weight. You will need to adjust your diet and exercise program.

Secondly, don't be discouraged if you don't see results right away. Weight loss takes time, so be patient when trying. Remember that even a small amount of weight loss can make a big difference to your health. A person carrying just ten pounds of extra weight places 40 pounds of pressure on their knees and other lower body joints. A buildup of fat in the body can also lead to inflammation as chemicals damage your tissues over time. One study showed that older women who lost at least 5% of their weight reduced their breast cancer risk by 12%.

Fat releases chemicals that make the body unresponsive to the effects of insulin, a hormone that maintains blood sugar levels. Losing just 5% of body weight reverses this effect.

Weight loss after 50 can be achieved safely and effectively with menopausal weight loss methods. With this book, you'll learn how to make healthy choices and lose weight sustainably.

Discover how metabolism and hormones change during menopause, and how to use this information to lose weight. Whether you want to drop a few pounds or achieve a significant weight loss goal, menopausal weight loss can help you improve your health.

You don't have to struggle to lose weight during menopause. When you have the right guidance, you can make healthy choices that will help you lose weight and keep it off. In this book, you'll find an overview of the best ways to lose weight for menopausal women over the age of 50.

Among the topics covered in the program are dieting for weight loss, exercise for weight loss, and staying motivated. The information you will receive will also teach you about the mistakes that menopausal women make when trying to lose weight. We highly recommend this book to anyone who wants to make a commitment to their health and wellbeing. But remember, change takes time. However, if you stick to a long-term weight loss plan, you will achieve your weight loss goals. Menopause Weight Loss Guide is the perfect resource for women over 50 who are looking to lose weight in a healthy and sustainable manner and wish to do so in a healthy and sustainable manner. Using this guide will provide you with simple, yet effective steps that will enable you to reach your weight loss goals. For better management of your menopause, you may also want to consult with your doctor or a menopause specialist. Managing hormones may require medical assistance. With the tips outlined in this guide, you'll be on your way to a healthier, happier you.

Chapter 1 - What is weight loss?

In order to better comprehend how weight loss and gain work, you may find it helpful to visualize your body as a balance of energy in and energy out. Your food provides you with energy, and you then burn this energy off during your daily routine - things like walking, shopping, and going to work. If you want to stay the same weight, your energy intake and output must be equal. You gain weight when you consume more energy than you need.

Weight loss is often the primary goal of many people when they decide to lose weight. It is necessary to burn more calories than you take in in order to lose weight. In order to do this, you need to eat less and exercise more.

Despite this, some people are still unable to understand what weight loss means because it isn't just about losing weight. It is also about adopting a healthier lifestyle that includes regular exercise, eating healthy meals, and making lifestyle changes to fit their needs. In this case, we are talking about a "lifestyle change.".

There are a few things menopausal women over the age of 50 have going for them when it comes to weight loss. Because of the health risks associated with being overweight during menopause, they are more likely to want to lose weight than younger women. Additionally, since they are no longer working and raising a family, they have extra time to devote to eating healthily and exercising.

What is metabolism?

Metabolism refers to the rate at which a body converts food into energy. It is affected by several factors, including the hormones produced by the body and the lifestyle choices made by the individual. By breaking down food, the body produces energy through metabolism, and when it does so properly, it produces energy as efficiently as possible. It can be described as the sum total of all the processes in the body that convert food into energy.

Steps to weight loss

Let's take a moment to recall a few things to keep in mind when trying to lose weight during menopause.

Beat your metabolism

As you age, your metabolism slows down. As a result, losing weight will be a little more challenging as you get older.

Combat hunger

In addition, your hormone levels may be changing, affecting hunger and appetite.

Focus on belly fat

Furthermore, menopause can result in changes in your body shape, which can make it difficult to lose weight in certain areas, such as the belly.

Step 1

It is important to start by understanding how menopause affects your body in the first place. You will learn about the changes in your metabolism and hormones, and how these changes can impact your weight loss efforts. Once you have a better understanding of how menopause affects your body, you can start making lifestyle and dietary changes to lose weight.

Step 2

The second step is to implement lifestyle changes that will help you lose weight. You will learn about the most effective exercises for menopausal women, and how to make changes to your diet that will help you lose weight. This means monitoring your progress and making sure you are losing fat, not muscle. You will also learn about the dangers of crash dieting and yo-yo dieting, and how to avoid these traps. You will also learn about the importance of getting enough sleep and managing stress, two important factors that can impact weight loss during menopause.

Step 3

The third step is to maintain your weight loss. This step will teach you how to keep the weight off for good, and how to prevent weight regain.

So, if you are a menopausal woman over the age of 50 who is looking to lose weight, know that it is possible.

Chapter 2 - What is Menopausal Obesity?

"According to an international study of obesity during menopause, nearly 39 percent of premenopausal women are overweight or obese."

For many women, menopause is a challenging process, but one of the biggest concerns they have is their weight. Your favorite pair of jeans may begin to fit tighter than they once did in your mid-to-late 40s, regardless of the occasional hot flash or mood swing that you may experience. You are not imagining this.

According to a landmark study, women gain about four and a half pounds during the transition to menopause in their 40s. A new review published in the journal Mayo Clinic Proceedings shows that women keep gaining about a pound and a half in their 50s and 60s.

Many women are unaware that changes in hormone levels can affect metabolism and appetite. This can cause many problems such as weight gain, loss of energy, and loss of libido.

The biggest problem with being overweight during menopause is the potential impact it has on your health. Therefore, as a woman experiencing menopause, it is important to lose weight for several reasons. Carrying extra weight can increase your risk of health problems such as heart disease, stroke, type 2 diabetes, and some cancers. It can also make it difficult to treat other symptoms that may already be present, such as high blood pressure and joint pain. Losing weight helps reduce the risk of developing these health problems and improve your overall quality of life. In addition, losing weight can relieve menopausal symptoms such as hot flashes and uneven mood.

Why do we gain weight after 50?

There are many factors that can cause you to gain weight after 50, including aging, hormonal changes, and lifestyle factors that increase your appetite. Menopause is a natural process that occurs when a woman's ovaries stop producing eggs and produce less estrogen as a result. Women's lives change significantly during menopause, a period of major physical and mental change. A woman's body shape may also change significantly when she goes through menopause as a result of hormonal fluctuations. The body is gradually storing more fat into the central portion, including the heart, and around the organs in the body. As a result, your shape may completely change into an "apple" rather than the "pear" or "hourglass" shape you desire. It is possible for this to happen even if you are not overweight. In addition, the pancreas may also be sensitive to the condition and may negatively impact blood sugar levels. Blood vessels that carry blood to the heart and brain can be damaged by high levels of blood sugar.

What role do hormones play in weight gain?

The levels of estrogen decrease during menopause, while the levels of androgen increase. It is believed that this hormonal imbalance affects energy balance by changing the signals that indicate hunger and satiety. A greater number of menopausal women will notice intense hunger signals, which will cause them to eat more, leading to an increase in weight during this time.

This often leads to women developing a "tummy", which often turns into an addiction to sugars and unhealthy fats, which their bodies will use to gain (estrogen producing) abdominal fat.

Estrogen

As a result of hormonal imbalances during the menopause period, abdominal fat is more likely to accumulate. Every single cell in your body is equipped with an estrogen receptor. Because of this, when estrogen levels begin to drop, your body will try to get estrogen from fat cells.

The hormone estrogen is involved in many different functions in the human body, such as controlling metabolism and blood sugar levels. When women reach menopause, their estrogen levels fall, which can lead to weight gain. Low estrogen levels and high androgen levels cause fat to be redistributed from the buttocks and thighs to the abdomen, resulting in the accumulation of abdominal fat. Combining low estrogen with high androgen levels results in difficulty losing weight and maintaining it.
The lower estrogen levels can lead to widespread joint pain, which is why many women reduce their daily exercise routine as a result of the lower estrogen levels. This can lead to weight gain during

menopause as well.

It is possible for low estrogen levels to cause the sympathetic nervous system to produce a "fight or flight" response. During this stress response, the stress hormones cortisol and adrenaline are also released. Due to adrenaline, the body can experience symptoms such as an increase in heart rate and breathing rate, dry mouth, and nervousness in the stomach, as cortisol releases glucose to increase energy to allow the body to escape danger. If there is no physical activity, this glucose triggers the release of insulin, which stores the glucose as fat. It is well known that stress causes "insulin resistance" and can lead to fluctuations in blood sugar levels. This increases your chances of developing two conditions namely diabetes type 2 and coronary artery disease.

Insulin

It is often believed that weight gain during menopause is caused by a decline in metabolism. It is, however, also possible that insulin resistance contributes to weight gain during this period. In the course of time, the body becomes less sensitive to its ability to respond to insulin and so the body becomes unable to utilize it to regulate blood sugar levels. In the event of insulin resistance, the body may start to store more fat which may lead to weight gain. It is also possible for insulin resistance to contribute to type 2 diabetes and other health problems as well. It is important that you discuss with your doctor whether insulin resistance is to blame for your inability to lose weight during menopause. The doctor will be able to order tests for your blood sugar and insulin levels so that he or she can recommend treatment if necessary.

Leptin and Adiponectin

The hormone leptin plays a vital role in the regulation of hunger and metabolism, as well as the processing of fat. It is a hormone produced by fat cells, and it works by sending signals to the brain to let it know when we are full. Losing weight typically increases the level of leptin in our body, which prevents us from overindulging. When women go through menopause, their leptin levels can drop abruptly, which can lead to a rise in hunger and weight gain.

The hormone Adiponectin regulates metabolism by helping to maintain the level of blood sugar in the body. Both of these hormones have been linked to hot flashes as well as subclinical insulin resistance. According to a study, women who had higher levels of leptin and adiponectin were more likely to experience hot flashes. An additional study found that women with higher levels of leptin and adiponectin were more likely to suffer from subclinical insulin resistance than those with lower levels of these hormones. Based on these studies, it appears that a link exists between these two hormones and both hot flashes and subclinical insulin resistance.

The two most common factors that lead to weight gain after 50 include an increased level of hormones that stimulate appetite (mainly ghrelin, a peptide released by the stomach), as well as a decrease in hormones that suppress appetite (most notably leptin, which is secreted by fat cells).

Ghrelin

The hormone ghrelin is also capable of influencing weight loss as it is often called the "hunger hormone" because it increases appetite. Among other things, our bodies produce less leptin, the hormone that tells us when we are full, as well as more ghrelin, the hormone which triggers our appetite. As a result, it should not surprise us that during menopause, we tend to eat more and gain weight. An increase in appetite, accompanied by an increase in body fat, is one of the consequences. Additionally, ghrelin affects other metabolic processes within the body, such as the release of insulin and glucose into the body. When you are trying to lose weight, keeping your ghrelin levels under control may be helpful to your weight loss efforts.

Testosterone

In addition to estrogen, testosterone is another important female hormone. In women who have large ovaries, decreased testosterone levels may result in a decrease in muscle mass and energy levels. So, eating exactly the same amount of calories as you did before menopause will result in a reduction of your metabolic rate.

Thyroid hormones

As a final note, thyroid hormones play a role in metabolism, and an imbalance in these hormones can make it more difficult for you to lose weight. It is important to note that thyroid hormones play an important part in the regulation of human metabolism, as well as the development of bones and muscles. As patients reach menopause, the production and supply of thyroid hormones are reduced, which can lead to low energy, fatigue, and excess weight gain.

HRT

A number of women complain that hormone replacement therapy (HRT) causes them to gain weight. You may find it more difficult to lose weight if you are over 50 and taking hormone replacement therapy (HRT). Women who take estrogen replacement therapy (HRT) may gain weight due to fluid retention (up to 10 pounds per month), although this is usually only a mild condition that will pass within a month or two.

There are several different types of hormone replacement therapy

(HRT) that can cause weight gain in women who are menopausal. A person who is taking combined estrogen and progestogen HRT tablets may experience an increase in appetite and fluid retention as a result of the medication. There is also the possibility of taking an estrogen-only HRT tablet, which can cause fatigue, making it difficult to exercise regularly. It is thought that injectable HRT and skin patches will cause less weight gain than oral HRT tablets, though they may still do so in certain women. It is recommended that you speak to your doctor about other options if you are on HRT and struggling to lose weight. In some cases, your doctor may suggest changing the dose or type of hormone replacement therapy that you are taking, or prescribing a different type of medication altogether.

Psychological changes

Menopause can also produce psychological effects such as weight gain-women often experience changes in their appearance due to aging, changes in their relationships, financial concerns, and fears about the health of themselves or their loved ones, among other factors. Moreover, the burden of caring for grandchildren and possibly due to brain fog can cause additional stress, which can lead to overeating and drinking to cope.

Women may also experience episodes of emotional eating from time to time. Emotional eating refers to eating in response to psychological triggers such as stress, worry, and anxiety. In the long run, emotional eating can cause weight gain and other health problems.

Chapter 3 - Ditch the diet

It's imperative for women experiencing menopause over 50 to avoid crash diets and yo-yo dieting. It is clear that these types of diets can be extremely dangerous for your health and can actually contribute to gaining weight. Women from all over the world have spent most of their lives yo-yo dieting, and it can be extremely frustrating to lose weight, only to regain it back even more. As such, restricting calories is an ineffective method of losing weight, as it ultimately reduces your basal metabolic rate.

It is true that many people lose weight and keep it off by restricting their food intake, but some find that this can lead to feelings of deprivation and a disinterest in food in the future. As a matter of fact, you may be even more likely to gain weight after losing it this way due to the fact that you've deprived yourself of the pleasure of eating. It is very important to continue to enjoy food as much as you did before you started losing weight in order to maintain your weight loss.

Instead of focusing solely on diet changes, make lifestyle changes that will help you lose weight in a healthy and sustainable manner. Getting enough sleep, eating a healthy diet, and exercising are all components of weight loss that are critical to your success.

Further, crash diets and yo-yo diets can also cause hair loss, fatigue, and irritability as well as causing additional health problems. It is critical to note that these are not just side effects - they can actually be a warning sign that something more serious is happening. If you experience any of these symptoms while you are dieting, you should stop immediately and speak with a physician.

When it comes to weight management, quick fixes can be misleading, especially when it comes to losing weight. In reality, there is no magic bullet that works overnight - these diets often result in long-term disappointment. We have found that a holistic approach to wellness will work better, with a healthy diet, regular exercise, and women being supported through their journey of self-discovery.

It is far more effective to make a couple of changes to your lifestyle to enable you to live a healthier lifestyle rather than to resort to drastic measures. If you want to live a healthier life, this is the best route to take.

If you are a woman who is going through menopause, you have enough things to worry about - don't add to the stress by trying to lose weight! Don't waste your time and money on fad diets and quick weight loss solutions that don't work long-term.

Fortunately, weight loss is easier today than ever before, with the introduction of the internet, as well as apps like MyFitnessPal, which can help you keep track of calories consumed and calories burned throughout the day.

How to lose weight without dieting

Having a healthy diet is an important part of losing weight, and there are some things that you can do to make sure that you're getting the nutrients you need. First of all, you should eat a balanced diet - you should aim for roughly 40% of your daily calorie intake to come from carbohydrates, 30% from protein, and 30% from fat. As part of your diet, you should also make sure that most of the calories you consume come from foods high in protein, healthy fats, and fiber.

If you are going through your menopause and you need to lose some weight, there are some foods that are particularly beneficial. Fruits, vegetables, and whole grains are some of the foods that are particularly beneficial. In general, it is recommended to stay away from processed foods and sweetened beverages.

In order to prevent any side effects of menopause, you should consume a balanced diet that includes the right quantity and type of vitamins, minerals, and other nutrients that are necessary to maintain healthy heart and bone health, as well as treat other menopause-related symptoms. Please note that the following is a summary and should not be used to substitute for a customized assessment by a specialist or for advice from your doctor or a menopause specialist.

Bump up your protein intake

Generally, the more protein you consume, the faster you will feel full. Compared to other foods, high-protein food has a higher filling capacity, so you will not feel hungry all day and you will have an easier time sticking to a healthy diet. Lean meats, chicken, fish, eggs, cheese, yogurt, legumes, and nuts are some examples of high-protein foods. Include at least once a week oil-rich fish such as salmon and mackerel in the diet. Use vegetable oils and spreads rather than animal fats such as butter. The product is an excellent source of unsaturated fats, including omega-3 fats, which are beneficial for your heart.

In addition to that, low-fat dairy products also provide a good source of protein. There is no doubt that the more protein you consume, the more calories you will be burning throughout the day. A recent study published in the Journal of the Academy of Nutrition and Dietetics reported that obese and overweight adults who consumed a higher amount of protein burned 60 more calories a day on average. This is especially relevant during menopause, during which protein consumption is of the utmost importance for the building of muscle mass and for preventing weight loss problems.

There is no doubt that muscle burns more calories than fat, so the more muscle you have, the more calories you will burn. Additionally, protein also plays an instrumental role in balancing your metabolism. In order to keep your metabolism working, it is helpful to eat foods that will help keep it functioning as we age. Consuming proteins may also help you control your appetite and help you feel full. Therefore, if you are menopausal, and you want to lose weight, you need to ensure you consume plenty of protein every day.

If you are a vegetarian or vegan, you should prioritize plant-based protein sources such as beans, lentils, and soybeans over animal protein sources. As an alternative to dairy milk and yogurt, choose low-fat dairy products and soy-rich plant-based alternatives.

Eat a whole-foods-based diet

The best way to lose weight long-term is to eat a diet that is based on whole foods. Diets are composed of whole, natural foods that are rich in vitamins, minerals, and antioxidants such as fruits, vegetables, whole grains, beans, nuts, and legumes. According to the findings of a recent study, women who consumed a minimum of two servings of fruit and vegetables a day were 29% less likely to become obese than people who consumed just one serving of fruit and vegetables daily. A number of starchy foods, such as potatoes, corn, and grains, have a low glycemic index and provide a body with a consistent source of energy.

Diets consisting of whole foods tend to be higher in fiber, and nutrient-dense, making them ideal for sustaining energy and keeping you satisfied for a long period of time. The fiber and nutrients found in these foods, as well as the low-calorie content, can help regulate your digestive system, thereby making you feel fuller for longer periods of time. Oats and barley: oats, oatcakes, oatmeal, pearl barley. These foods provide certain types of cholesterol-lowering fiber. This means that you are less likely to overeat and gain weight. Whole grains are also a good source of nutrients, so they will help you to stay healthy as you lose weight. A diet that emphasizes whole foods is often lower in refined grains and added sugars, which can be beneficial to your health and weight loss.

Try out intermittent fasting

Intermittent fasting is a good option for weight loss during menopause because it helps to regulate hormones. When you fast, your body is able to rebalance hormone levels and reduce inflammation. This can lead to weight loss and increased energy levels. Intermittent fasting is also beneficial because it helps to improve digestion and promote detoxification. If you are menopausal and struggling to lose weight, talk to your doctor about whether intermittent fasting is right for you.

Eat less at night

Eating less at night is good for weight loss during menopause because it helps to regulate your hormones. Eating less at night can help you lose weight. A study of 28 women found that a reduced nighttime diet, which recorded a total of 3,600 calories per week, resulted in a weight loss of 1.7 kg (3.7 pounds) in 12 weeks.

When you eat late at night, your body has a harder time digesting the food. This can lead to hormone imbalances that cause weight gain. Additionally, late-night eating can disrupt your sleep patterns. This can lead to fatigue and overeating during the day. If you are trying to lose weight during menopause, it is best to eat your last meal of the day at least 3 hours before bedtime.

Limit added sugars

Sugar is bad for weight loss during menopause because it is high in calories and low in nutrients. It will cause you to gain weight and can also contribute to health problems such as diabetes. If you're struggling to lose weight and you're concerned about your calories from added sugar, you may want to reduce the amount of sugar you consume in your diet. Read the food labels - avoid products with too much sugar or artificial sweeteners. Avoid using diet sodas and other sugar-laden beverages. Try drinking water or a sugar-free beverage instead. When you're dining out, choose low-sugar drink options like fruit juices.

Hydrate

If you have a tendency to eat when you're not hungry, hydrate! It's a common mistake to mistake thirst for hunger. Thirst is a surprisingly common reason why we snack when we're not actually hungry. Have a glass of water before you reach for a snack or put it away altogether, and wait for hunger to strike.
Water is an important part of a healthy and balanced diet. It helps to keep your body hydrated, which is important for overall wellbeing. It also helps to maintain the digestive system, and the immune system, and aids with blood pressure regulation.

Some studies suggest that drinking water can also help burn calories. In a 2014 survey, 12 people who drank 500 ml of cold room temperature water experienced increased energy consumption. They burned 2-3 percent more calories than usual in the 90 minutes after drinking water. Water can also temporarily increase the body's resting energy expenditure or the number of calories burned at rest.

Avoid coffee

While coffee can be a great way to jump-start your day, but if you're trying to lose weight and burn fat, go easy on the caffeine — especially in the afternoon, as it can leave you dehydrated and cause sleep issues. As mentioned earlier, lack of sleep increases hunger hormones. All of these things lead to weight gain.

The less caffeine you consume, the better. Although consuming little to no caffeine can feel initially devastating, you'll soon find that a lack of jittery side effects and boosted energy levels will make it easier to get going in the morning. When it comes to caffeine, it's best to gradually wean yourself off your favourite drinks.

Moderate alcohol intake

Some women find that they become less tolerant of alcohol during menopause. That might be the time to take a good look at your drinking habits — alcohol is harmful for many reasons, and it might be contributing to the symptoms you've been experiencing. Alcohol is often high in sugar and empty calories (there are approximately 130 calories in a 5-ounce glass of red wine). Sugar content will trigger an insulin spike, followed by low blood sugars.

You should moderate your alcohol intake for a few reasons. First, alcohol is high in calories and can cause you to gain weight. Second, alcohol can disrupt your sleep patterns, which can lead to weight gain. Third, alcohol can worsen menopausal symptoms such as hot flashes and night sweats. fourth, you might be tempted to drink to quench the dryness, but alcohol also slows the metabolism, meaning your fat stores are more likely to be used up. Alcohol can have a number of other negative effects on the body, including a decrease in testosterone (in both men and women) and an increase in cortisol. So it's important to moderate your alcohol intake if you want to lose weight during menopause.

Improve your gut health

Improving gut health has hugely beneficial effects on mood, weight and sleep, to name just a few. There are many resources online that discuss gut health, including books, podcasts and videos, but you should always consult with your doctor. We know how important it is to consume a variety of fruits and vegetables. A ratio of approximately 2 pieces of fruit to 8 portions of vegetables is recommended. Researchers have found that this variety promotes a healthy gut and may help reduce symptoms such as constipation and bloating. Check out online guides on 'eating the rainbow', which encourages us to include many different colors of fruit and vegetables in our diet. By doing so, a variety of micronutrients are ingested, which are essential for good health.

Choose the right supplements

There are a number of supplements that can help with weight loss, and menopausal women may find them especially helpful. The most common natural supplements for weight loss in menopausal women are green tea and grape seed extract. Green tea is a diuretic (meaning it increases the production of urine) and grape seed extract is a mild antioxidant. Both of these supplements can help you lose weight by increasing metabolism, which is the rate at which your body uses energy. There are a few different supplements that can help with weight loss during menopause. One is black cohosh, which can help to regulate hormones and ease menopausal symptoms. Another is Vitamin D, which can help to improve metabolism and bone health. Finally, omega-3 fatty acids can help to reduce inflammation and promote heart health. Talk to your doctor about which supplements are right for you. They can also help you figure out the best dosage.

Chapter 4 - Control your daily habits

Menopausal women often complain about having sleep issues and stress. This can significantly impact your metabolism and prevent you from losing weight. Controlling stress, getting enough rest, and stopping smoking can help aid weight loss and reduce your risk of illness.

Stress

Stress can have a big impact on weight loss during menopause. When you are stressed, your body releases the hormone cortisol. Cortisol can lead to increased appetite and cravings for unhealthy foods. It can also cause your body to hold onto fat instead of burning it for energy. If you want to lose weight during menopause, it is important to find ways to manage stress - a major factor in preventing weight loss. Try deep breathing exercises, meditation, and journaling - all great ways to reduce stress. Seek out support from friends and family if you are feeling overwhelmed. Making time for yourself and doing things that make you happy can also help reduce stress levels.

Improve your sleep quality

Sleep difficulties are common during menopause. Hot flashes, night sweats, and stress can all lead to difficulty sleeping. It's also possible that sleeping difficulties are connected to weight gain as a result of hormone imbalance and appetite problems during menopause.

If you are having trouble sleeping, try to establish a regular sleep schedule. Go to bed and wake up at the same time every day. Avoid caffeine and alcohol before bed. Create a relaxing bedtime routine. Exercise during the day to help you sleep better at night. If you are still having trouble sleeping, talk to your doctor about possible treatments.

Stop smoking

Cigarette smoking is one of the worst things you can do for your health. It increases your risk of lung cancer, heart disease, and stroke. It also causes wrinkles and premature aging. If you are menopausal and struggling to lose weight, quitting smoking is one of the best things you can do for your health. Not only will you lose weight, but you will also feel better and have more energy. Cotinine is also a by-product of smoking. Cotinine is a metabolite that can lead to increased levels of insulin and leptin, both of which may cause weight gain.

Chapter 4 - How to exercise for weight loss

Exercise not only helps to boost your metabolism, but it also helps to keep your bones and muscles strong. There are many different exercises that can help with weight loss during menopause, but some are more effective than others. A combination of cardio and strength training is the best way to lose weight during menopause.

Walking, running, and swimming are great cardio exercises for burning calories and losing weight. Strength-training exercises like lifting weights or using resistance bands can also be helpful, as they help to build muscle and boost metabolism. Yoga and Pilates are also beneficial for managing menopausal symptoms like hot flashes and mood swings. Try to do at least 30 minutes of cardio and 20 minutes of strength training 3-5 times per week.

Ultimately, the best exercise for weight loss during menopause is the one that you enjoy and will stick to in the long term. Talk to your doctor or a personal trainer if you need help getting started.

As we age, our bodies change and lose muscle mass. This process is called sarcopenia and it can start as early as age 30. After menopause, women lose muscle mass even faster. As a result, we need to be careful when exercising during menopause. Over-exercising can lead to injuries and make it harder to lose weight. Instead, focus on moderate exercise that will help you maintain your muscle mass and lose fat. Try to get at least 30 minutes of exercise most days of the week. Walking, biking, swimming, and yoga are all great options.

How to burn belly fat?

It's almost always true that excess weight piles up in your thighs and hips when you're young, but as you get older it seems to accumulate in your stomach as well. This can cause some frustration when you have to adjust to a new body type that was different from the one you had in the past. It is possible to lose some belly fat during menopause by doing certain specific things. Combining cardio and strength training is the best way to lose fat during menopause. Make sure that you do at least 30 minutes of cardio and 20 minutes of strength training at least 3-5 times per week. You can also do exercises such as pilates and yoga to tone the muscles in your stomach and feel less bloated.

Weight training or walking instead of high-intensity exercises can help you lose weight. Over a period of three months, you will lose belly fat and gain strength if you replace spin class, boot camp, and HIT cardio with resistance bands, weights, and walking. The purpose of exercising is to balance and optimize insulin and cortisol levels. In addition to increasing insulin sensitivity, resistance training allows the pancreas to better control blood sugar levels by improving insulin sensitivity. The pancreas will eventually produce less insulin as a result. With insulin carrying less fat over time, the body must mobilize accumulated fat for energy production. Exercises with resistance are slow-burning exercises that take a long time to build up to a certain level. By strengthening your muscles, you are increasing their metabolic activity. Consequently, you burn more fat, and as a result, your metabolic rate is increased.

Make sure you are not at risk for osteoporosis

In addition, as a woman ages and her estrogen levels decline, she is no longer able to maintain or build as much bone mass as she did in the past. It also means a woman is at greater risk of developing osteoporosis. As the name suggests, osteoporosis is a condition that causes the bones to become brittle and weak with age. The condition afflicts approximately one-third of all women over the age of 50, particularly after they have gone through menopause. There are a number of reasons why certain types of exercise may not be the best option for you if you have osteoporosis. The reason for this is that exercise can place additional strain on already fragile bones that are already under strain. As a result, fractures or other types of injuries may occur. It is also important to mention that a lot of exercises involve high-intensity activities, such as running or jumping. These activities can also result in fractures or other injuries in women who suffer from osteoporosis. Additionally, some exercises may require you to use weights or other equipment that you may find difficult to use if you have osteoporosis.

Even if you suffer from osteoporosis, it is still important to stay active and to exercise regularly. It is advised that you avoid activities with high impact and exercise with due care when using weights or other equipment. For advice on the type of exercise that would be suitable for you, please consult your doctor.

You should not give up on losing weight just because you are going through menopause. You will be able to reach your weight loss goals if you work hard and stay motivated. By experimenting with different exercises, you can find a routine that works for you.

Chapter 5 - Get additional weight loss support

Prescription Medication

During menopause, some medications can be prescribed in order to assist with weight loss. It is very likely that your doctor will prescribe hormone therapy for you to help balance your hormones and reduce the symptoms of menopause. Furthermore, they may also prescribe a weight loss drug such as Semaglutide (Wegovy) or the more common prescription weight loss drugs such as liraglutide (Saxenda), naltrexone bupropion (Contrave, Mysimba), orlistat (Alli, Xenical).

The medications that are listed above tend to work in unique ways and may suppress your appetite, increase your metabolism, or discourage the absorption of fat by your body. As a rule, doctors only prescribe if the patient has a BMI of 30 or higher, or at least 27, and has conditions that can be worsened by weight gain, such as type 2 diabetes or high blood pressure.

Liraglutide

A weight-loss injection known as Liraglutide (also known as Saxenda) is available for women going through menopause who wish to lose weight. This helps to curb your appetite and cravings so you will eat less and lose weight as a result. Saxenda is a prescription medication, so it's very important that you discuss it with your doctor if you are considering taking it.

Naltrexone bupropion

Naltrexone bupropion, more commonly known as Contrave in the United States and Mysimba in the EU, is an FDA-approved prescription-only weight-loss drug that has the ability to increase your metabolism and help you lose weight. This product works by increasing the rate of metabolism and decreasing the appetite by acting on the hypothalamus, which is the part of the brain responsible for regulating the body's appetite, temperature, and energy expenditure. The use of Contrave should only be done under a doctor's guidance.

Orlistat

In addition to the many weight loss medications on the market, Orlistat is one of the most common. It works by delaying the breakdown of fat in the small intestine, therefore reducing the amount of fat absorbed by the body. By reducing the amount of calories absorbed from food, you will be able to lose up to 5% of your body weight in the process. It is important to consult your physician before deciding whether or not to take Orlistat.

In addition to these medicines, you will have to maintain a proper diet and exercise regimen in order to control your weight. Your doctor may also recommend a low-calorie diet or other lifestyle changes to help you lose weight. Even though it might be difficult for you, it is possible to lose weight during menopause if you put your mind to it.

Hormone replacement therapy

There are a variety of ways in which estrogen can be replaced by estrogen-replacement therapy (HRT) to assist women who are undergoing menopause to lose weight. In general, estrogen has been proven to help boost the metabolism, which in turn can lead to weight loss. In addition, estrogen could also help to suppress appetite, which is another factor that contributes to weight loss. And last but not least, estrogen plays a role in the breakdown of fat cells. This is one-way fat cells can be broken down, making it easier for people to lose weight. It is important for menopausal women who are trying to lose weight to know estrogen is a powerful hormone that can be of substantial help to them. Please speak to your physician if you are thinking about starting any hormone therapy since there are many risks and side effects of estrogen therapy. Many doctors do not recommend hormone therapy to every woman. Instead, they recommend that women try to lose weight by exercising and dieting, rather than relying on hormone therapy.

Another option for weight loss during menopause is hormone injections. These can be given by a doctor and help to regulate your hormones. This can make it easier to lose weight, as well as ease other menopausal symptoms. If you are interested in this option, talk to your doctor to see if it is right for you.

Chapter 6 - How to maintain your weight loss

It is not always easy to maintain your weight loss, especially if you are trying to lose weight in order to lead a healthier lifestyle. Even for those who have lost significant amounts of weight as a result of a weight loss diet or exercise routine, maintaining their weight loss can be quite a challenge. Keeping weight loss is a constant battle, and most people who successfully lose weight will find that they gain weight back much faster than they initially lost. Therefore, maintaining weight loss is all about avoiding gaining weight back. In order to maintain weight loss, you need to continue to make healthy food choices and exercise. It is also important to monitor your weight and body fat percentage regularly. Here are some tips on how you can stay motivated and committed to your weight loss goals:

- Maintain a food journal - this will allow you to keep a closer eye on how you eat on a daily basis and make sure you aren't eating more than you need - it will help you avoid making unhealthy decisions in the future.
- If you have a goal weight in mind, write it down so you do not forget what you are striving for in the future.
- Set your own goals - how much weight do you aim to lose in the first week? How about the following week?
- Identify the reasons why you were able to lose weight and stay motivated in the future. If you use these reasons to motivate yourself in order to continue living a healthy lifestyle, then you can use them as triggers.
- Scheduling your meals and snacks ahead of time is a great way to make sure you stay on track with your diet.
- Don't skip meals - skipping meals can throw your body's metabolism out of sync. This will cause you to crave unhealthy foods more often.
- Don't skip your workouts - a little exercise every day will

keep your metabolism going and thereby help you stay on track with your weight loss.

- Stay physically active - the more active you are, the more calories you burn and the easier it is to maintain your weight.
- Get a fitness buddy - Exercising with a friend can be a great way to keep you motivated to stay on track with your goals.
- Work on creating a healthy lifestyle habit that you can sustain over time such as making healthy eating choices when you get home from work or designing a new exercise routine that you can stick with.
- Make your weight-loss goals realistic and don't get discouraged if you lose weight and then gain it back.

Conclusion

In the last chapter of this series, we will explain how your life will be different after you've lost your target weight. We will also share some parting advice with you. In addition to the physical changes, there are many reasons why menopause can affect women's health. These reasons include not only the emotional ones but psychological ones, too. The majority of these problems can be alleviated or improved by losing weight, which is a fantastic way to improve your general health and well-being, as well as your quality of life.

Most of us know how difficult it is to lose weight. You will likely struggle for a long time to reach your primary weight goal. In the end, though, you can feel a lot better about yourself once you have lost a healthy amount of weight. The following are some of the physical benefits you can expect once you have lost weight:

- More energy - you should feel a lot more energetic after losing weight.

- Strength - you will be stronger and be able to lift more weight.
- Better posture - you should have a better posture than you did before.
- Happiness - you should be happier and more confident than you were before.

In such a unique time in your life, it's important to surround yourself with positive and supportive friends and family members, as well as a community of women who have the same goals. Don't be afraid to share what you are doing with your family and friends. It will come as a surprise to you how motivating it can be when you have friends and family cheering you on. You can help yourself stay on track by asking a close family member or friend to join you on your journey — who can be a great source of inspiration, motivation, and encouragement while you're going through it.

Menopausal women over 50 who follow the techniques outlined in this book for weight loss may expect to lose weight and improve their overall health. In the long term, exercise and nutritious eating will help them reduce weight. Furthermore, they will benefit from improved heart health, reduced risk of osteoporosis and other age-related disorders, and increased mood and energy levels.

The best way to lose weight is through a healthy diet and regular exercise. You may also need to discuss hormone therapy or other treatments to treat menopause symptoms with your doctor. If you are dedicated, you can lose weight.

It is our hope that following the weight loss instructions on this mini-guide can help menopausal women over the age of 50 to live a healthier, happier life.